Kesias Garba Djikoloum

Fetal alcohol syndrome

Kesias Garba Djikoloum

Fetal alcohol syndrome

A threat to women in sub-Saharan Africa

ScienciaScripts

Imprint

Any brand names and product names mentioned in this book are subject to trademark, brand or patent protection and are trademarks or registered trademarks of their respective holders. The use of brand names, product names, common names, trade names, product descriptions etc. even without a particular marking in this work is in no way to be construed to mean that such names may be regarded as unrestricted in respect of trademark and brand protection legislation and could thus be used by anyone.

Cover image: www.ingimage.com

This book is a translation from the original published under ISBN 978-613-8-44125-0.

Publisher:
Sciencia Scripts
is a trademark of
Dodo Books Indian Ocean Ltd. and OmniScriptum S.R.L publishing group

120 High Road, East Finchley, London, N2 9ED, United Kingdom
Str. Armeneasca 28/1, office 1, Chisinau MD-2012, Republic of Moldova, Europe
Printed at: see last page
ISBN: 978-620-6-18827-8

Table of contents

Dedication:

I dedicate this book to my mentor, Dr Hamadou Djibo, head of the public health department, teacher-researcher and lecturer at the Faculty of Health Sciences at Abdou Moumouni University in Niger. One of the best professors at the Niamey Institute of Public Health in Niger. His humility, dedication and availability are legendary.

Please accept my gratitude.

Thanks

I would like to express my gratitude to all those who contributed to the production of this book.

Book summary

Fetal Alcohol Syndrome (FAS) has been the subject of extensive hospital research in Chad. A little-known disease in sub-Saharan Africa. A real threat to children's survival. Premature deliveries, debilitated children, abortions, low birth-weight babies, various types of malformations and stillbirths are cases often encountered in our maternity wards. Had we taken the trouble to investigate the causes? Although alcoholism in pregnant women is not the only cause, it does contribute to increasing the rate of these pathologies, which constitute a permanent, lifelong handicap. Only prevention can save the lives of these innocent victims.

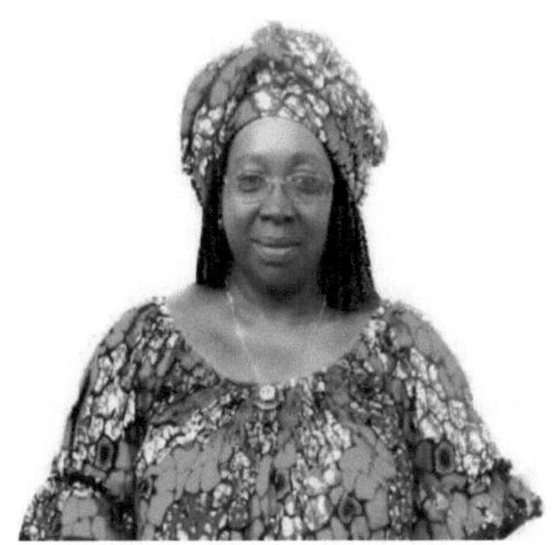

Biography: Kesias Garba Djikoloum was born on April 15, 1963 in Koyom, East Mayo-Kebbi, Chad. For the past 40 years, she has been fighting against mortality and morbidity in mother-child relationships. She holds a post-graduate diploma (DESS) in reproductive health from the Niamey Institute of Public Health in Niger. She is married and has five (5) children.

INTRODUCTION :

Alcohol is an old product, as old as the world. Traditionally and industrially prepared from cereals, fruit, sugar cane, honey, dates and other ingredients, alcohol remains a danger, even a scientifically known poison, for many organs. Before looking more specifically at alcohol consumption by pregnant women and the risks it entails for the fetus and child, it is important to review the general facts about alcohol.

First of all, alcohol consumption is a socio-cultural phenomenon that very often accompanies the most significant events in our lives: a wedding, a birth, a birthday, community work or a christening. Alcohol is also perceived as an element of joy and pleasure, but also of unhappy events such as bereavement, divorce, arguments, failure and loneliness. That's why it's hard to look at alcohol consumption solely in terms of its harmful and dangerous effects. And yet, given the physical and psychological impact of alcohol abuse, it also represents suffering and anguish. If the dangers of alcohol consumption concern everyone who uses it, they are all the more serious for women.

Women, once the guardians of good morals, now rival men in their consumption of alcohol.

These days, alcohol consumption among women is taking on worrying proportions.

In Africa, for example, only elderly women were allowed to drink discreetly at social events.

Nowadays, women of all ages publicly indulge in alcohol consumption. Rural women are particularly prominent at weekly markets and betting sales, where alcohol flows freely all night long, competing with their smurs in the cities. However, it's important to know that alcohol consumption among women has consequences for reproductive health. Not to talk about it is to maintain the population's ignorance on the subject. Prevention is therefore essential.

First and foremost, it should be pointed out that very few epidemiological surveys on female alcoholism have been carried out in French-speaking Africa. Nevertheless, the reports of three surveys carried out in Chad illustrate this reality.

According to the WHO 2011 report, Chad is a country where alcohol consumption by adults is high and rising: 19% of women over the age of 15 drink alcohol, compared with 23% of men **(1).**

The study on alcohol consumption and food security carried out in July 2012 in Chad by Djikoloum Magourna of the Chadian Blue Cross, in rural areas one in three alcohol consumers is a woman **(2).**

The EDS-MICS (Demographic and Health and Multiple Indicator Survey) report in Chad 2014-2015 ,39% of women aged 15 and over consume alcohol in Mandoul and Mayo-kebbi. In Moyen Chari and Tandjilé this percentage is 36% and 34% respectively. **(3)**

-In the past, women's alcohol consumption received little attention from researchers and the WHO, because it was considered a taboo subject, and because women drinkers felt marginalized and guilty, but this is no longer the case. Indeed, women's mentalities have evolved, and the major risks run by female consumers have led to the breaking of the silence.

- In fact, women react differently to alcohol than men. For the same weight and quantity of alcohol, a woman's blood alcohol level is 20% higher than that of a man. Women's livers are much more sensitive to alcohol, as their bodies contain less water than men's. This is a factor in the risk of alcohol poisoning. This makes women more vulnerable. **(4)**

Not only does the woman's body tolerate less alcohol, but she also induces Fetal Alcohol Syndrome (FAS) in her unborn baby. We also know that not every alcoholic woman is likely to give birth to a child with FAS. Genetic and physiological factors may influence the risk. We are also certain that the handicap caused by alcohol is irreversible. Unfortunately, this syndrome is little known among women, and even among health personnel in Chad.

Fetal Alcohol Syndrome (FAS) was the subject of our research work at the Institute of Public Health in Niger in 2014, and we propose to publish the present book to enlighten the public in general, women of childbearing age, pregnant women and their babies, public health students and health personnel in particular, as this important public health problem cannot resolve itself if no intervention is undertaken.

This awareness-raising work would have a positive impact if governments decided to implement the recommendations made by the author of this book.

This book is divided into four parts:

1- Alcohol and pregnancy

2- Fetal alcohol syndrome in Chad

3- SAF prevention in Chad

4- recommendations

Part 1

I-ALCOHOL AND PREGNANCY

What is fetal alcohol syndrome?

Fetal Alcohol Syndrome (FAS), also known as alcoholic embryo-fetopathy, refers to the consequences of alcohol intoxication of the embryo or fetus during pregnancy, disrupting the development of its organs and causing malformations and lifelong disabilities.

Severe alcohol intoxication of the fetus results in growth retardation, malformations and, above all, brain damage, with major cognitive and behavioral disorders.

In other words, FAS is a disabling and irreversible pathology caused by the mother's alcohol consumption during pregnancy.

It is the most frequent congenital anomaly after trisomy 21. FAS is a real public health problem.

On the one hand, it constitutes violence to the embryo or fetus during its life in the womb (a real violation of the child's rights before birth), and on the other, an irreversible handicap for the child after birth.

These children have difficulty being self-sufficient. They suffer from stunted growth, unstable behavior and lower IQs. It is acknowledged that most of them are unable to feed themselves and learn to care for themselves at the same pace as other children born normal. In a country like Chad, where social care is a problem, these children do not socialize, and are a social and economic burden for their parents.

1.1- DISCOVER SAF

Fetal alcohol syndrome was first described in France in 1968 by French pediatrician Paul Lemoine.

Having observed a number of identical-looking newborns in incubators, in 1958 he began a study of children of alcoholic mothers, based on observation of 127 children from 62 alcoholic families. In 1968, Paul Lemoine et cool..., described for the first time the clinical picture of children suffering from the syndrome in Nantes, France. These findings were published in the journal Ouest Médical under the title "Les enfants de parents alcooliques: anomalies observées à propos de 127 cas".

At the same time, West Coast researchers Smith, Jones and Streissguth published their findings, similar to those of Paul Lemoine, under the title Fetal Alcohol Syndrome.

In French literature, the pediatrician Philippe Dehaene suggested in 1995 the term "syndrome d'alcoolisme fmtal" (fetal alcohol syndrome): "He justifies this by the fact that the fetus is not an alcoholic, but has passively undergone his mother's alcoholism.

1.1.2- Prevalence of FAS worldwide

After its discovery in France and the USA, FAS was confirmed in Canada, Reunion Island and South Africa.

In North America, FAS affects 1 to 3 children out of every 1,000 live births;

(5)

-In Canada, approximately 1% of the population is estimated to be affected by FAS, and 280,000 Canadians are affected, particularly in the rapidly growing northern community (6).

In France, it is estimated that fœtal falcoholism spectrum disorders affect 1%, i.e. 7,000 new children every year.

Around 500,000 French people suffer from alcohol-related after-effects (ARF) to varying degrees. **(7)**

FAS itself is the leading cause of non-genetic psychomotor retardation in France. According to Dr Damblin in a 2010 survey, 7,500 children are born each year in France with a damaged or malformed brain.

-On Reunion Island, the annual incidence of FAS is very high: 4 to 8 children per 1,000 live births, with 1% of these children placed in specialized institutions for mental retardation**(8).**

-In South Africa, the rate of FAS is the highest in the world, according to a study by Denis Viljoen. It is estimated at 57 cases per 1000 newborns.

This is because some women may be abusing poor-quality alcoholic beverages to deliberately harm the health of their future babies in order to collect disability benefits**(9).**

These FAS children are often a social burden, requiring lifelong specialized care. This serious and confirmed syndrome is carefully screened and studied in paediatric wards in many developed countries, while it is ignored in sub-Saharan countries, including Chad. Yet this syndrome is a major handicap for young children. With this in mind, we set out to conduct a study on this delicate and taboo subject.

With regard to our country, Chad, a research study on FAS was carried out by Ms. Djikoloum Kesias on the **"epidemiological and clinical characteristics of Fetal Alcohol Syndrome (FAS) in three hospitals in Ndjaména, Chad"**: Hôpital mère enfant, Hôpital de l'Union, Hôpital Notre Dame des Apôtres, the results of which confirm the existence of FAS in our country.

1.1.3- Pathophysiology of alcohol in pregnancy

Pregnant women who drink alcohol endanger the life of their fetus.

Ingested alcohol rapidly passes into the bloodstream, then reaches the embryo or fetus via the placenta by simple diffusion. One hour after absorption, alcohol levels are equivalent to those of the mother.

The alcohol then passes into the liver of the immature fetus, which does not yet have its own degradation systems. This results in the following effects caused by alcohol absorption.

At the organogenesis stage, there is a decrease in the fmtus in utero due to :

- reduced blood circulation and spasm of placental vessels.

-A slowdown in the process of cell division in the embryo;

A deficit in synaptic contact establishment and nerve melanization;

ischemia and spasm of the placental vessels result in hypo-perfusion of the embryo and/or fetus;

-Stunted growth of the fetus in utero and reduced cell division during organogenesis promote malformation of various organs.

As for a dose-effect relationship or threshold dose, numerous studies clearly state that we don't know the dose of alcohol below which there is no risk for the baby. What's more, it's certain that alcohol is not useful for the baby's development.

In the fully manifested form, fetal alcohol syndrome includes pre- and post-natal growth retardation, delayed psychomotor development, learning difficulties at school, character and behavior disorders, craniofacial dysmorphia and intellectual deficits. The consequences of fetal alcoholism are certainly serious, but if the mother stops drinking, the risk diminishes significantly.

Alcohol has a teratogenic effect in other so-called atypical forms, i.e. likely to cause different types of congenital malformations, as well as numerous cases of babies dying a few days after birth, reduced fetal weight during pregnancy and after birth, premature deliveries and repeated abortions often wrongly attributed to chromosomal aberrations due to a lack of research.

1.1.4- Risk factors

-Exposure frequency

Prenatal exposure to alcohol is a risk factor for abnormalities at all stages of pregnancy. The questions raised by this risk are: is there a dose and a period when this risk is nil? Are there alcoholic beverages whose consumption has no effect on the fetus?

The dose-effect or threshold dose relationship varies widely according to various studies of daily and regular consumption:

Increased malformative risk: daily consumption of more than 6 glasses (Ernhart, 1987);

IUGR: daily consumption of three glasses, or 1 to 2 glasses (Larroque, 1993).

Lower IQ: for 2 drinks/d or more (Stresissth, 1989)

All studies point to a threshold weekly dose below which there would be no disorders: 7 glasses:

Alcohol consumption equals :

- Acute drinking has more harmful consequences than regular, daily drinking (Stresisst, 1989).

Threshold value to be modulated according to certain individual embyofetal sensitivities (Jacobson, 1994), among which the child's genotype seems to have a predominant importance (Sokol, 1980).

Nature of social and family environment: offspring of alcohol-dependent mothers from disadvantaged backgrounds more affected (Bingo, 1987).

Period of drinking and consequences:

SCHEMATICALLY :

Day 1: may prevent the egg from implanting;

Between the 3rd and 4th week: minor consequences on the skull and certain parts of the embryo's face;

Up to week 7: May split palate and lips

1^{e} quarter

-Craniofacial dysmorphia;

-Organ, muscle and skeletal damage.

2eme and 3eme quarter:

-Worsening of hypotrophy

(Fetal growth slowed dramatically)

-Behavioural problems ;

-Mental retardation ;

On the central nervous system (CNS)

1er trimester: severe disorganization

2nd trimester: heterotopias; cortical dysgenesis; significant effects on motricity and likelihood of spontaneous abortion;

3rd trimester: white matter destruction lesions.

France, America, Canada and WHO recommend zero risk and total abstinence from alcohol consumption during pregnancy.

As far as the exposure period is concerned, any consumption at any time can have an effect on the fetus.

Smoking and poly-drug addiction :

Tobacco and other drugs associated with alcohol represent a very high risk for the fetus: not all alcoholic women are likely to give birth to a child with FAS. This risk is also a function of certain individual embryo-fetal sensitivities (Jacob Son; 1994). Among these, the child's genotype seems to be of paramount importance (Sokol, 1980).

-Nature of social environment: if the alcoholic mother comes from a disadvantaged background and spends a large part of her life there, she may give birth to an FAS child (Bingo; 1987).

1.1.5- Saf diagnostics

-Growth retardation ;

-Characteristic dysmorphia ;

-Microcephaly;

-Organ malformations ;

-Central nervous system (CNS) abnormalities.

Saf in children (1)

-Craniofacial disorders ;

-Growth retardation ;

-Malformations ;

-Neurobehavioral aspects.

Saf in children (2)

Face :

-Narrow eye slits ;

Collapsed nasal bridge, hook-shaped tip, eversion of nostrils

-Middle stage hypoplasia

elongated, convex watch-glass philtrum ;

-thin, narrow upper lip ;

Small, recessed chin;

-Third eyelid (epicanthus);

-Hypertelorism;

-Persistence throughout childhood and adolescence.

Neurobehavioral aspects

- ➢ **Impact on intelligence quotient (IQ)**

  - ✓ FAS is recognized as a major cause of retardation

  - ✓ Stability of IQ over time

- ➢ **Consequences for activity and attention**

- ✓ They are too lively, incessantly restless, impatient and distracted (Lemoine 1968).

- ✓ Hyperkinetic disorders

- ✓ Attention deficit

  - ➢ **Consequences for memory**

  - ✓ Deficits in auditory and spatial memory.

Evolution and fate of adult saf.

-Intellectual retardation

-Behavioral disorders

-impulsivity, instability, hyperactivity,

-Psychopathological disorders: sleep disorders,

-Emotional disorders :

-Alcohol and/or drug dependence **(10)**

1.1.6- Classifications and dysmorphia

  - ➢ Some classifications are based on dysmorphia according to P. Dehaene:

✓ **FAS type 1:** children with one or two characteristic dysmorphic features;

✓ **FAS type 2:** children with all 4 signs of dysmorphia

SAF characteristics :

-narrowing of the palpebral fissures ;

-crushing of the root of the nose and turning up of the tip;

-philtrum indistinct and convex ;

-hypoplasia of the lower jaw.

✓ **FAS type 3**: children with severe caricature dysmorphia associated with :

-growth retardation

-a reduction in head circumference of at least 2.5 standard deviations (Sempé and Pedron curves)

-several other malformations.

✓ **FAS type 4:** children of alcohol-dependent mothers with suspected dysmorphic features at birth, without subsequent confirmation (type 4 corresponds to the fetal alcohol effect (FAE) of American and Canadian authors) **(11).**

1.1.7- Differences between FAS and FAE (Fetal Alcohol Effects)

FAS is the most serious condition, the easiest to diagnose, but also the least common.

FAE is a more widespread, more subtle, partial disease that is harder to diagnose.

Part 2

1. Fetal Alcohol Syndrome in Chad

These are essentially the results of our DESS research work in reproductive health on the epidemiological characteristics of fetal alcohol syndrome in three hospitals in Ndjamé na in Chad from in 2013 at the Niamey Public Health Institute in Niger.

1.1- Sites surveyed

The Mother and Child Hospital, the Union Hospital and the Notre Dame des Apôtres Hospital are the three health establishments included in our study, and here is a synoptic table of their profiles.

INFORMATION GENERALE	HOSPITAL MERES ET CHILDREN	HOPITAL DE L'UNION	THE HOSPITAL NOTRE DAME APOTRES
Geographical location	Quartier Gardolé au N'Djamena Center	Chagoua south of N'Djamena	Chagoua south of N'Djamena

Creation date	Created in 2010	Created in 1999	Created in 1948
Objectives	Fighting mortality and morbidity mother and child	Decentralize basic health care in order to bring the population of health service	Taking care of all sick people without racial distinction ethnicity and religion
Services	-Birth room -Pediatrics -Neonatology	-Birth room -Pediatrics	-Room for birth -Pediatrics
How it works	-24h /24	7.30 a.m. to 4.30 p.m. + day-care service	8 a.m. to last patient+on-call service

Doctor	-2 Full-time physicians 2 Physician assistants	-1 Head physician -1 Assistant doctors	1 Head Physician -1 Assistant doctors
Midwife	-5 SFDE -1 supervisor	-3 SFDE	-2 SFDE
Nurse	-3 IDE -1 IDE	-2 IDE -1 IDE	-2 IDE
Dirty boy	-1 garcon de sale	-1 dirty boy	-1 dirty boy
Dirty girl	-1 dirty girl	-1 dirty girl	-1 dirty girl

The criteria that guided the choice of these sites were :

-Geographical location

-Socioeconomic characteristics of mothers attending these hospitals.

A total of ninety-four (94) mothers were studied.

1.2- SOCIO-DEMOGRAPHIC PROFILE OF SAF MOTHERS

Table I: distribution of mothers in the three hospitals in the city of Ndjamena according to age in 2013.

Age	Frequency	Percentage
15-19 years	16,0	17,0%
20-24 years	**33,0**	**35,1%**
25 -29years	23,0	24,5%
30 -34 years	13,0	13,8%
35-39 years	3,0	3,2%
40-44 years	6,0	6,4%
Total	**94,0**	**100,0%**

The 20-24 age group is the most represented, with 35.1% of women surveyed.

If we exclude the 25 to 29 age group, this represents a total of 59.6% of our sample, or just over the majority of mothers surveyed. In other words, most of the FAS mothers in our study were between 25 and 29 years of age.

Table II: Distribution of mothers in the three Ndjaména hospitals according to their marital status in 2013.

Marital status	Frequency	Percentage

Single	13,0	13,8%
Divorced	1,0	1,1%
Bride	**80,0**	**85,1%**
Total	**94,0**	**100,0%**

The table above shows that 85% of the mothers surveyed, i.e. around 9 out of 10, are married.

Tables III: distribution of mothers of children according to their professions in the three Ndjamena hospitals in 2013.

Profession	Frequency	Percentage
Retailer	*20,0*	21,3%
Student	**32,0**	**34,0%**
Civil servant	16,0	17,0%
Housekeeper	21,0	22,3%
Other	5,0	5,3%
Total	**94,0**	**100,0%**

The table above shows that 34% of mothers are pupils/students. They are followed by housewives, who account for 22.3%.

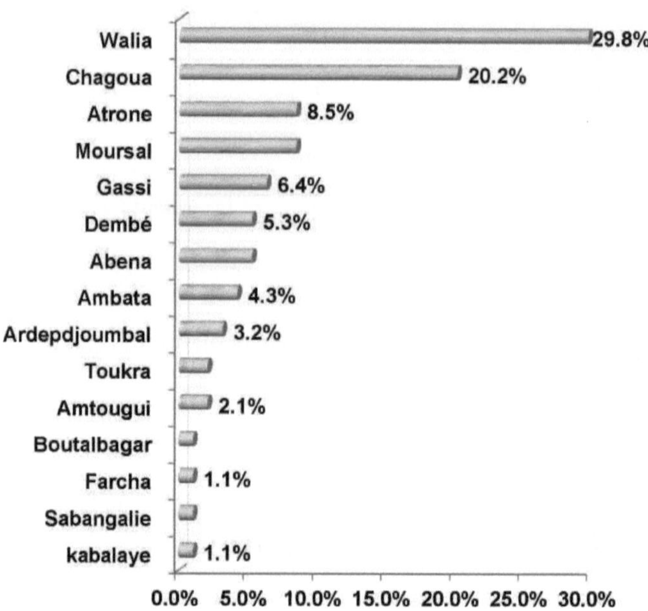

Figure 1: distribution of surveyed mothers according to their provenance in 2013.

The figure shows that 29.8% of mothers come from Walia and 20.2% from Chagoua. The other districts are poorly represented.

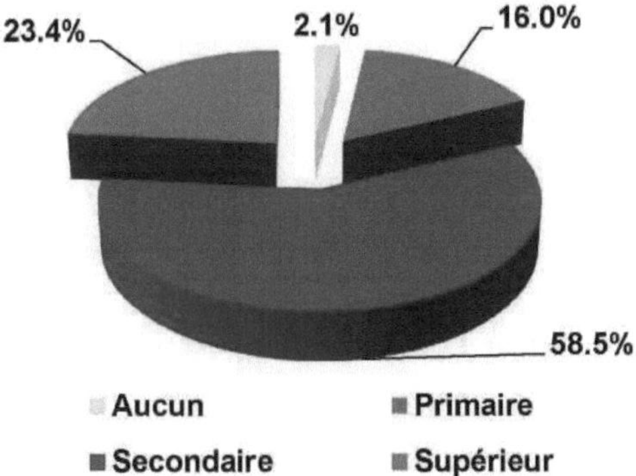

Figure2: distribution of mothers surveyed in the three Ndjamena hospitals according to their level of education in 2013.

According to the figure above, 4 out of 5 mothers (75%) have at least secondary education, and only 2% of mothers surveyed have no education, i.e. they can neither read nor write.

In short, most of the mothers surveyed were very young, under thirty (30).

In conclusion, most pregnant women are married. In terms of professional occupation, the majority are either students or housewives, i.e. lacking adequate financial resources. 50% of these mothers also live in Walia or Chagoua: two neighborhoods where alcohol consumption is very high.

Table IV: Distribution of children according to whether or not they have FAS at three Ndjamena hospitals in 2013.

1.1.3- Prevalence rate

SAF	Frequency	Percentage

	Frequency	Percentage
Without SAF	86,0	91,5 %
With SAF	8,0	8,5%
Total	**94,0**	**100%**

The above table shows that **91.5%** are FAS-free, with a prevalence rate of :
8.5% among children born to surveyed mothers.

Table V: Distribution of children in the three Ndjaména hospitals according to type of FAS.

SAF	Frequency	Percentage
Typical SAF	2,0	25 %
Atypical SAF	6,0	75%
Total	**8,0**	**100%**

We can see from this table that one (1) child in four (4) has typical FAS.

Table VI: Distribution of surveyed mothers of children by type of alcohol consumed in the three Ndjaména hospitals.

Alcohol	Frequency	Percentage
Traditional	3,0	3,2 %

Modern	**50,0**	**53,2%**
Both	41,0	43,6%
Total	**94,0**	**100%**

53.19% of mothers who drink alcohol regularly have

More than half, 53.2%, have consumed modern alcohol.

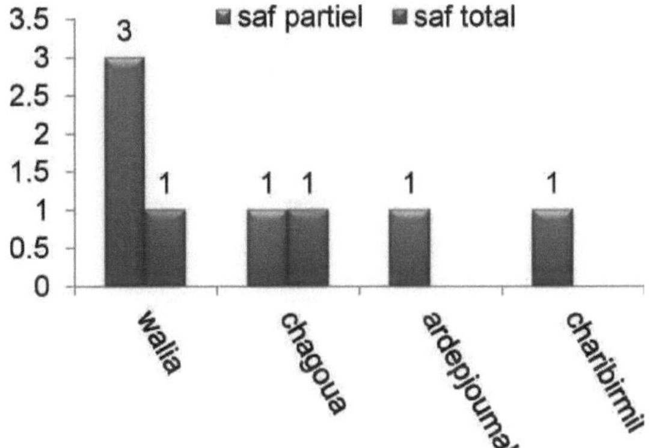

Figure3: FAS distribution by neighborhood. It's easy to see that one child in 2 with FAS comes from Walia.

We can see from this table that children with typical FAS come from Walia and Chagoua.

Different clinical types of fretal alcohol syndrome according to gender.

Table VII: Distribution of FAS cases by sex of child.

Gender	SAF atypical	Typical SAF	Total
M	4,0	1,0	5,0
F	2,0	1,0	3,0
Total	6,0	2,0	8,0

We can see from this table that more than half the children with FAS are male.

Table VIII: Distribution of FAS cases recorded in the three Ndjaména hospitals according to the mother's age in 2013.

Age range	Partial SAF	SAF Total	Total
15-19	1,0	0,0	1,0
20-24	1,0	1,0	2,0
25-29	2,0	0,0	2,0
30-34	1,0	1,0	2,0
35-39	1,0	0,0	1,0
Total	6,0	2,0	8,0

Children whose mothers were under 30 had more FAS than those whose mothers were over 30.

Table IX: Distribution of FAS by type of alcohol consumed

Type of alcohol	Atypical fetal alcohol syndrome		alcoholTypical fetal alcohol syndrome		Total	
	Case	%	Case	%	Case	%
Local	0,0	0%	0,0	0%	0,0	0%
Modern	2,0	25%	0,0	0%	2,0	25%
Both	4,0	50%	2,0	25%	6,0	75%
Total	6,0	75%	2,0	25%	8,0	100%

We can see from this table that three(3) children out of four(4), or 75%, come from mothers who have consumed both(2) types of alcohol.

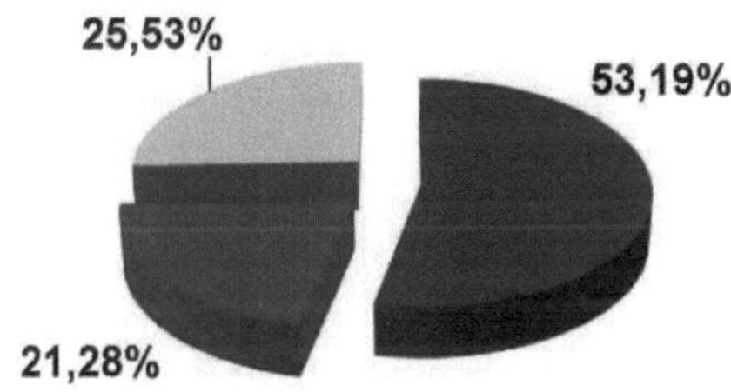

Figure 4: Distribution of mothers by frequency of alcohol consumption.

1.1.4- Results from a questionnaire administered to healthcare staff.

Table XIV: distribution of staff surveyed in the three Ndjaména hospitals according to their category in 2013.

Category	Workforce	Percentage
Doctors	3,0	30%
SFDE	5,0	50%
IDE	2,0	20%
Total	10,0	100%

One in two (2) of the staff surveyed at the three hospitals was a midwife.

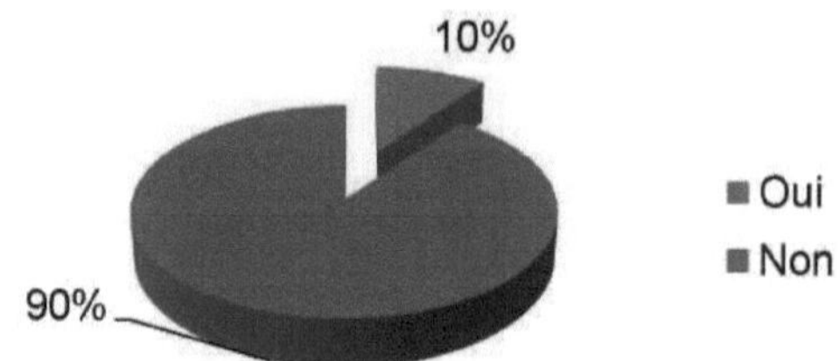

Figure 5: Breakdown of staff by knowledge of FAS

The figure above shows that little is known about FAS by the healthcare staff surveyed at the three Ndjamena hospitals. One health worker in 10 is aware of FAS. In sum (90%) of healthcare staff are poorly informed. This lack of knowledge about FAS among healthcare staff is a threat in this field.

1.1.5- Determinants of alcohol consumption by mothers during pregnancy.

In the majority of cases, women have become alcoholics as a result of following in the footsteps of their friends and husbands. Some women deliberately consume alcohol for the following reasons: to deliver a baby with a clear complexion, vigorous, intelligent and clean, without caseosa varnish on the skin at birth, as caseosa varnish, a natural substance to protect the baby, is interpreted as being the husband's sperm (impure). To avoid shame, tradition forbids women in pregnancy, especially at term, to have sexual relations. Another reason, according to our survey, is that alcohol also promotes abundant milk secretion after childbirth.

This mistaken belief about alcohol leads some mothers to abuse local alcohol or industrial beer during pregnancy, creating a vicious circle of transplacental consumption between mother and child. These children are already born alcoholics, even if they show no signs of FAS. At birth, the baby reacts in an unusual way, becoming agitated when the cord is cut, due to the effect of the addiction.

Part 3

1. How can we combat FAS in Chad?

1.1-Women

> Primary prevention

- Raise awareness of the dangers of alcohol among girls of childbearing age and pregnant women, as the December 2013 survey shows that 100% of women are unaware of this pathology.

-May the woman who gives life also be able to protect that life.

-Encourage women to take part in FAS information sessions.

-Work with pregnant women on false rumors by giving them accurate information.

> -secondary prevention

-Systematic screening for FAS from birth for babies born to mothers known to be alcoholics, so that the necessary advice can be given.

> Tertiary prevention: support and follow-up for the mother and baby born with FAS; care for the FAS baby;

Part 4

I-Recommendations.

Based on the results of our study, we make the following recommendations:

To the Ministry of Public Health

- ✓ Numerous studies have recognized and confirmed that FAS leads to permanent and irreversible disability in both children and adults, so given the serious nature of this pathology,

- ✓ We recommend the following:

- ✓ Organize a mass awareness campaign with the media throughout the country;

- ✓ integrating FAS research into alcohol policy in Chad ;

- ✓ vote for a law on alcohol during pregnancy;

- ✓ To provide technical and material support to associations working to combat alcoholism in Chad;

- ✓ That the Ministry of Health allocate the necessary resources for such research.

- ✓ Introduce an alcohol module in health and social care training schools;

- ✓ Create a medical-social action center for FAS children:

- ✓ Train qualified personnel for systematic screening and appropriate care of FAS children (dysmorphologists, speech therapists, psychotherapists, psychoeducators, physiotherapists).

Hospitals:

- ✓ Make mothers aware of the consequences of alcohol consumption during pregnancy during prenatal visits.

- ✓ Strengthening the Focused Prenatal Consultation (**CPNR**)

- ✓ Organize educational sessions on alcohol consumption before any treatment for pregnant women.

- ✓ Train midwives to provide specialized counseling for pregnant women.

To the Ministry of Education

That maternal alcohol abuse be integrated into the family life education program and taught in schools to all girls of childbearing age.

FOR MOTHERS :

Organize awareness campaigns to make pregnant women aware that life is sacred and that they have the right to protect it:

Conclusion:

At the end of our study of the epidemiological and clinical features of Fetal Alcohol Syndrome, FAS is very real indeed. If nothing else, it's a public health problem that can't be solved on its own unless action is taken.

BIBLIOGRAPHIC REFERENCES

1. (WHO report 2011 in Chad) Speech by the Minister of Health on the workshop to validate the draft law against alcoholism in Chad 2012.

2. Djikoloum Magourna .D. Chad Blue Cross study on security in Chad in 2012.

3 .2014-2015 EDS-MICS (Demographic, Health and Multiple Indicator Survey) report for Chad Accessed on o4- july-2022 at 00h30mn

4. Books consulted: vade-mecum d'alcoologie page 32, **and J-C.Archambault**, A. Chabaud page 42. July 04 -2022 at 00h41mn.

5. **Jones, kl and Smith,D.W. Recognition** of the Fetal Alcohol Syndrome in Early infancy, lancet no 2,1973,P.999-100

6. **Paul L. J.-C.Archambault**, A. Chabaud édition Masson: Alcoologie ; alcool et grossesse Page 12

7. **Streissguth, A.P.**Fetal Alcohol syndrome. A Guide for families and committees, Baltimore (Maryland), Paul H.Brookes publishing company.1997Health *Canadawww.*sc-hc. ge.*caconsult June 5, 2014 at 7:30 p.m.*

8 **-Dr** **Damblin.D.9**, rue Victor Hugo-97450 Saint Louis0692709433/0692820618 Email: coeurdereseau@reunisaf.com in 2008Consult June 27, 2013 at 9:00 pm

9. **Denis** V. http://www.contrepoint.org/2013/14/111285-Afrique-du-sud-syndrom-d'alcoolisation.consulted on 27/06/2013www.wsws.org.consulté

10. **Observatoire Régional de la Santé**: Repère sur le syndrome d'alcoolisation fœtal e(SAF) à la réunion.http://runisat.comconsulté April 13, 2013

11. **Dehaene** L'alcool et la grossesse, presse universitaire de France (PUF) Que sais - je n⁰ 2934, janvier 199555

Observatoire français des drogues et de toxicomanie Institut des recherches scientifiques sur les boissons. April 2012 consult June 05, 201

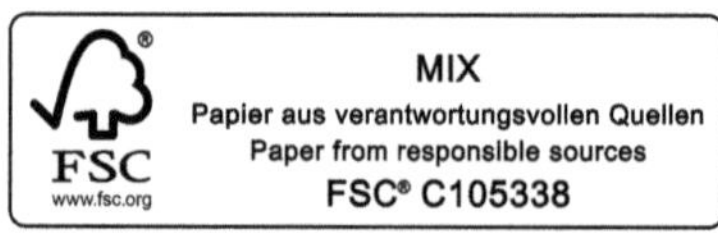

Printed by Books on Demand GmbH, Norderstedt / Germany